FAT BLASTING SMOOTHIES

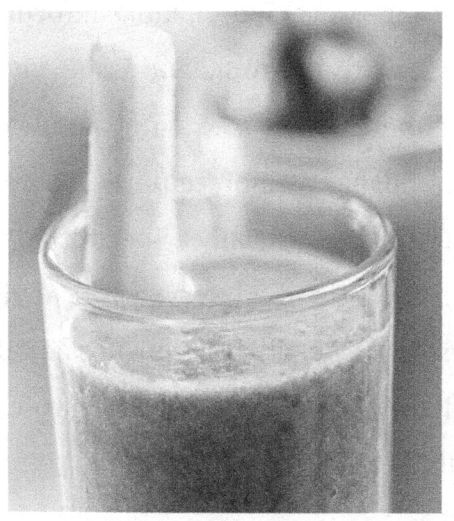

10 Day Smoothie Cleanse – Lose up to 14 Pounds in 7 Days

By

Jason Lee

Copyright 2015 by Content Arcade Publishing - All rights reserved.

This document is geared towards providing exact and reliable information in regards to the topic and issue covered. The publication is sold with the idea that the publisher is not required to render accounting, officially permitted, or otherwise, qualified services. If advice is necessary, legal or professional, a practiced individual in the profession should be ordered.

- From a Declaration of Principles which was accepted and approved equally by a Committee of the American Bar Association and a Committee of Publishers and Associations.

In no way is it legal to reproduce, duplicate, or transmit any part of this document in either electronic means or in printed format. Recording of this publication is strictly prohibited and any storage of this document is not allowed unless with written permission from the publisher. All rights reserved.

The information provided herein is stated to be truthful and consistent, in that any liability, in terms of inattention or otherwise, by any usage or abuse of any policies, processes, or directions contained within is the solitary and utter responsibility of the recipient reader. Under no circumstances will any legal responsibility or blame be held against the publisher for any reparation, damages, or monetary loss due to the information herein, either directly or indirectly.

Respective authors own all copyrights not held by the publisher.

The information herein is offered for informational purposes solely, and is universal as so. The presentation of the information is without contract or any type of guarantee assurance.

The trademarks that are used are without any consent, and the publication of the trademark is without permission or backing by the trademark owner. All trademarks and brands within this book are for clarifying purposes only and are the owned by the owners themselves, not affiliated with this document.

TABLE OF CONTENTS

Introduction 7

Chapter 1: How To Use This Book 18

Chapter 2: Starting Out 30

    Fruits and Seeds: 35

    Vegetables: 44

    Others 48

    Equipment 50

    Things to Note 55

Chapter 3: Action Plan 61

Chapter 4: Fruit-based Smoothies 71

Chapter 5: Vegetable based Smoothies 81

Chapter 6: Energizing Smoothies 91

Chapter 7: Breakfast Smoothies 101

Chapter 8: Quick Smoothies 110

Conclusion 118

INTRODUCTION

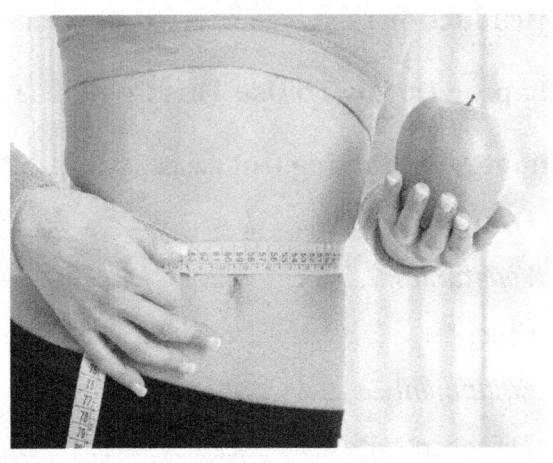

Do you need a body makeover? Do you wish to shed those flabs without going through that dreadful cardio? Or do you simply want to feel *great* about your body? If your answer is YES, then look no further, you are reading the book that will help you transform your body and *blast* away the layers of unwanted fats in less than HALF a month. In this book, you will learn step by step actionable plan to cultivate a refreshing 10 day smoothie body cleanse diet that not only makes you feel great but lose some pounds as well.

The book will explain in detail the benefits of a smoothie diet, how the smoothie diet works and the things you need to get started.

You will also be given an extensive list of delicious recipes to follow. I will also include detailed action plans to guide you in maximizing the potential of this awesome list of recipes.

Now, I know what you are thinking – is this the real deal or just an over-hyped book. Is this just another book that dumps a bunch of data on me and leaves me on my own? Well, the short answer is no, but allow me to explain further.

I used to be just another girl, slightly overweight, a little low in self-confidence and just living my life, without the slightest care for my body. I would gorge on crackers and ice cream whenever I want and I would never put on a pair of skinny jeans (not that I can fit anyway), let alone go near a pair of bikinis.

It was until one morning that I looked into the mirror and I realized that if this carries on, I would never have the chance to look beautiful in my life. In fact, it is not only about looking beautiful, I wanted to have something to look forward to; I wanted to prove that I *could* achieve something.

To overcome this, I spent hundreds of dollars going after the next diet pill, the next slimming lotion and the next beauty product. I was deeply seduced by their promise of beauty and perfection that I was willing to part with a good chunk of my fortune on it without a second thought.

Every time I bought something, I told myself that this is the *one*. Well, of course it never was.By at the end of the year, I literally looked the same and felt the same. I was lethargic and burnt out from the countless hours spent on the Internet researching the next magic pill.

I knew that I had to take real substantial action to improve my situation. I needed to do some serious reflection on what is going on.

I gradually come to the realization that there are actually no magic pills. There is no shortcut to the healthy lifestyle and looking great. Because *think about it* – If this solution exists, *everybody* will be going for it. And yet, why is everybody still searching for it?

It was then that I read about the science of cleansing the body and was immediately intrigued by this idea. There is no chemical pills you have to eat, everything is organic and if the legend is true, you can lose weight in a relatively short time. So I took action in my life and changed my diet. I went on a month long smoothie diet plan, severely cut down on the carbohydrate intake from my life and starting to work out to boost my metabolism.

And wow, the transformation was *instant.*

Not entirely in the physical sense, but mentally, I felt that I'm less lethargic and negative. Every morning when I woke up, I felt fresh and recharged and I wanted to keep going. I felt much better than when I was chasing the next diet pill behind a computer screen, reading the likely fake reviews generated by outsourced workers.

Well, through my years of research, I was finally able to conclude that if you want to lose weight, you have to do the below 3 points correctly.

1) Conviction
2) Diet
3) Exercise

If you are currently reading this, I do not doubt your conviction, good job! This leaves us with exercising and dieting. Yes, I agree that exercising is important (and I highly encourage it) but truth be told, many of us simply HATE it. That feeling after we ran 15 miles or did 200 hundred burpees just doesn't appeal to many of us.

If this is an excuse (which it should not be), you are left with your only choice, that is to fix your diet. We have to eat everyday anyway, so why not eat something that both healthy and delicious so that our bodies are treated with the proper nutrients they require?Why not go on a smoothie diet?

You might ask - why should I go on a smoothie diet plan?

The number one reason for drinking smoothie (besides losing weight) is that it cleanses and detoxifies the body. There are many factors that contribute to weight gain, and the one that is often overlooked is excess toxin in the body! During exercise, if your body is overloaded with toxins, it will be unable to function at its maximum efficiency to burn away calories. If the body does not have enough energy to burn calories, fats will not go away! If you consistently feel bloated, constipated, experience low energy level/fatigue, headache or chronic pains, it is a sign that your body contains toxin that are not effectively removed.

The most effective weight-loss programs should focus on both fat loss and detoxification, which lead to overall improved health and wellness. Raw greens can heal the body. You will detoxify your body through elimination of certain foods for ten days and reprogram your taste buds to desire healthy, nutrient-rich foods. After you complete the cleanse, you will never have to count calories or do expensive meal plans again,

As your body get acclimatized to the greens and unprocessed food, it will naturally crave and desire healthy foods in the future.

In the following chapters, I will explain what EXACTLY is the smoothie diet, how to hit the ground running and create an actionable plan. You will also understand important things to note when you are on the diet, how to keep yourself motivated and disciplined to see through the plan. You will also be given an extensive list of great fat blasting recipes to last you through the 10 days and beyond!

If this sounds good for you, let's get started!

Chapter 1: How To Use This Book

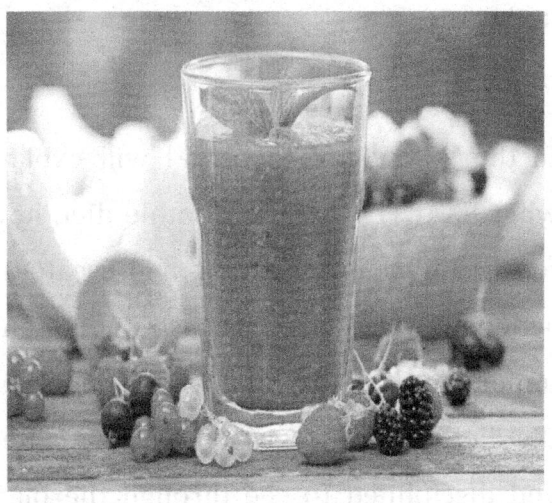

I spent a lot of effort putting this book together so before we go any further, I urge you to really have the same motivation and conviction to implement and execute what is taught in this book. If you feel that giving up your soda, pizza and fries is too hard to achieve, there really is no point reading on and you might as well seek a refund. If you want to read on, that is great! I hope that you will stick with what I have to say and let me show you what is possible with the 10 day smoothie cleanse.

What exactly is a smoothie anyway? How is it different from juicing? Why should we drink smoothie instead of just doing the regular diet of salad and fruits?

Many are often confused by the concept of juicing and smoothie and think of them as the same thing. No, they aren't!

Juicing: Juicing involves a process where the natural liquids, vitamins, and minerals are extracted from raw fruits and vegetables, this process strips away any solid matter from the fruits and vegetables and you're left with liquid only. This liquid isn't just your regular liquid of fruit juice or vegetable juice; it is packed to the brim with the vitamins, minerals, anti-inflammatory compounds, antioxidants, and phytonutrients in a single glass of goodness. Juicing is a great way to consume the best nutrients from fruits and vegetables without having to chow down on a bunch of solid greens and fruits! Our bodies will absorb the nutrients very quickly and efficiently because the body doesn't have to break down anything. The juice is completely void of any fiber and this enhances the digestion process.

Smoothie: Now, a smoothie involves the blending and blitzing of the entire food product into a thickened slush. Every part of the fruit and vegetable is added to the mixture with the exception of the skin and the seed. Smoothies are great as the fiber from the fruit provides sustenance, filling your stomach up and it gets your bowels moving. With making a smoothie, nothing is wasted and you consume every part of the raw food.

So why should you go for smoothies instead of juices? First of all, we don't like food wastage, if you can; try to consume the raw food in its entirety. Those aside, here are 5 good reasons why smoothies are beneficial:

1) Smoothies Are Whole Food – A smoothie is still a whole food because they are packed with fiber, minerals and tons of nutrients. Juices, on the other hand, are not whole foods. The reason is because the fiber has been removed, and this potentially removes a lot of nutrients that are attached to the fiber. Fiber is a critical aspect of digestion and we do not want to remove it directly from our diet. If you are on a juicing diet, you probably have to buy extra vegetables to consume just the fiber.

2) Faster to Make – For those of you who claim that you have no time to exercise, you probably will prefer a smoothie because it takes a much shorter time to make than juicing. I can simply pop in a banana, half an apple and stuff some a bunch of kale and watercress in my blender and 30 seconds later; I'm drinking a smoothie. There are also fewer cleanup stepsinvolved with smoothie because of the simplicity of it. A juicer must be disassembled and scrubbed clean before being kept back on the shelf. The whole process is just more troublesome for you busy bees.

3) Smoothies Fuels Your Body– If you are looking to maximize the potential of your body cleansing diet, you will want to exercise frequently. Personally, I love running and smoothies consistently provide me with fuels on my runs.Juices, on the other hand, do not provide the same lasting fuel provision as smoothies because the fiber has been removed. Without fiber to contain the juice and liquid, juices gets digested much faster and quicker. Juices also lack in protein, which is why it may leave you feeling hungry the entire day after a work out session. Coincidentally, the perpetual feeling of hungriness also leads to snacking which is in fact counter – productive to what you are trying to achieve!

4) Blended Green Smoothies Oxidize Slower Than Juices - It is often advised to drink a juice as soon as possible after making it. This is because juices are highly susceptible to oxidation because of the way they are being made and concocted. Experiments have shown that juices oxidize much faster than smoothies. Once your juice has oxidized, you begin to loose the goodness that is contained within the liquid and it will not taste as fresh anymore. Smoothies on the other hand are able to last through prolonged storage.

5) Green Smoothies Are A Sustainable Dietary Habit - Smoothies can serve as an actual meal. You can swap out your breakfast; lunch or dinner for a smoothie every single day because it contains EVERYTHING you need to live a healthy lifestyle. Juicing, on the other hand, feels more like a snack rather than a meal. At times, it feels more like a beverage rather than a proper hearty meal feeling a smoothie can provide. The thick paste-like texture of a smoothie helps it taste like a proper solid food as well.

So, what exactly causes you to lose weight by going on a smoothie diet? The answer is quite simple. Fats are what they are because the body has taken in more energy than it needs to expend. Hence, the energy is converted to fats and stored in the body until it needs to be used. All the processed food you consume plays a part in this role because they are refined and much easier to absorb than whole food. This, in turn, induces you to eat more because since the food gets digested faster, you feel hungry more frequently.

As a result, your body takes in more energy than it needs. Processed foods are usually unhealthy and are modified to taste "nice" so that we become more receptive to it. Think candies, white rice, spaghetti and burritos etc.

On the other hand, when you are on a smoothie diet, your body will feel full all the time because smoothies are fiber packed. You are also supplying your body with a steady stream of nutrients that the body needs, hence making you feel great. At the same time, the food that you blended in a smoothie does not contain a lot of carbohydrates (which becomes sugar once you've consumed them) and fats. This in turn greatly minimizes the amount of energy you consume every day. If your body is expending more energy than it is taking in, it has to get energy from somewhere else and guess what - it acquires the energy by burning fats from all over your body, and that, is why you slim down during a smoothie diet!

Of course, one can argue that isn't it better to not just eat anything at all? Sure, but prolonged starving will lead to host of other medical issues such as abdominal and gastric cramps. Furthermore, you are starving the body of nutritional minerals and vitamins it needs function properly as a system. With a smoothie diet, not only do you get to enjoy something that tastes great, you are also consuming lesser energy for your body to burn than your average daily diet.

The book is broken down into the preparation phase and the actual course of action phase. Make sure that you educate yourself completely in the preparation phase before moving to the actual course of action. You should have the necessary knowledge on which ingredients your body needs, as well as the necessary tools and equipment to get started. In the course of action phase, you will be given a complete daily routine of the 10-day plan; you will be taught the best ways to consume your smoothies and some important things to note when you are on the smoothie diet.

To make the full use out of this book, follow the action plan recommended here and do not deviate from it too much. It is important to stay disciplined to see the best results.

Chapter 2: Starting Out

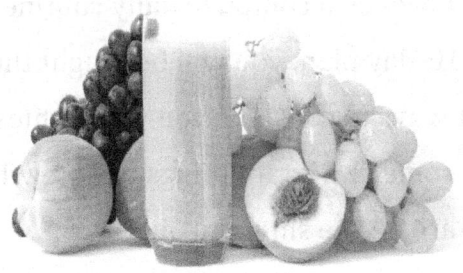

Now that you are well aware of the advantages of smoothies and how to maximize the potential of this book, let's get on with how you should prepare for the start of the smoothie plan! There are a few things that you need to be aware of before you embark on this exciting journey.

Fat blasting smoothies

Firstly, you need to adjust your mentality, you are switching your diet completely and you need to stay convicted to this path. If you give up after 2 days, it becomes pointless.

Secondly, you have to be aware of the variety of options out there for you to consume. In a nutshell, you need a crash course on the variety of ingredients that is out there.

Thirdly, you need to have the equipment to make your smoothies. You cannot make a smoothie with just a pair of knife and fork!

This chapter will teach you just how you should get started.

Mindset

For all you junk foodies out there, this is going to be a pain and I will not sugar coat it. Going through a diet of veggie and fruit slushes will not make you feel good initially because you will not be accustomed the sudden in take of raw, organic whole food. You may feel some churning in the stomach and a little bit nauseous to begin with. Go through the first two days and you should start to feel better. What is more important during this period of time is to stay motivated to your cause. You are turning your life for the better and shedding those POUNDS. Nobody said it was going to be easy and you definitely should not be expecting it. Find someone to talk to or find some form of support if you really require it. Your parents, spouse or friends are always there for you. If you are already a natural vegetable lover to start with, this is going to be a breeze and I believe you will be in love with smoothies by the end of this journey. It is yet another interesting and easy way for you to consume what you already love.

Once you are in the right mindset, you are ready to move on to the next point.

Ingredients

Ingredients are what that is going directly into your stomach. Knowing your ingredients will provide you with the knowledge to make healthier smoothies. With that knowledge, you can be creative to do make anything you want. Now, the variety of greens and fruits are many, I will highlight a few that I feel are staples to the smoothie diet so that you can get started straight away after reading.Feel free to look up more ingredients from the Internet if you are keen to find out more.

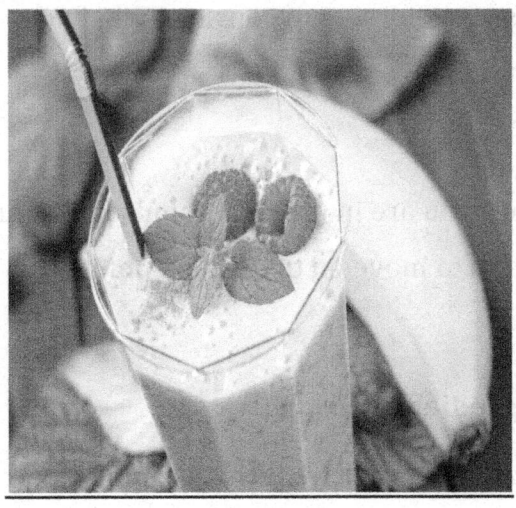

FRUITS AND SEEDS:

Apricots: On acalorie-for-calorie basis, apricot actually contains more of potassium than banana, which is pretty amazing for such a humble fruit. Dietary potassium can lower blood pressure by countering the adverse effects of consuming sodium. A potassium-rich diet also helps to reduce the risk of developing kidney stones and it also helps to decreasebone loss.

Blueberries: Blueberries are truly a condensed nutrient packed "pill", delivering very high amounts of vitamins, fiber, and phytonutrients like quercetin and ellagic acid. The last two compounds may protect against chronic diseases including cancer and heart disease.

Quercetinis also a hot topic in the sports nutrition world because of anti-inflammatory and other health benefits. Blueberries are also found to contain one of the richest sources of proanthocyanidins. These phytonutrients decrease free radicals levels that are directly linked to aging!

*Cranberry:*Cranberry juice provides a tart taste along with powerful flavonoids called proanthocyanidins. Research shows drinking cranberry juice cocktail daily can promote urinary tract health, providing protection against certain harmful bacteria that cause urinal tract infections.Cranberry juice can also help to lower the risk of heart related ailments and assist in sustaining cardiovascular health.

Grapes: Red wine, which is made from grapes, provides antioxidant resveratrol that protects you from heart diseases. By adding red or purple grapes or grape juice to your next smoothie, you'll take in compounds that can help reduce blood pressure and cardiac hypertrophy, lower levels of low-density bad cholesterol, and slow the progression of hardening of the arteries.Grapes are very effective in overcoming and eliminating constipation.

Pomegranate: Pomegranate juice is greatly beneficial to your health, particularly on the heart. Itkeeps the arteries flexible and decreasing the inflammation in the lining of the blood vessels. It reduces the potential risk of clogging in the arteries. Artery congestion can cause a restriction in the flow of blood to the heart and brain. The high amount of dietary fiber, both soluble and insoluble in pomegranate also helps to improve digestion and regulate bowel movement. Since it has no saturated fats or cholesterol, it is highly recommended for those aiming to lose weight.

Soy:Long relied upon as the go-to protein by vegetarians and vegans, soy can be of benefit to all athletes. Besides offering a host of vitamins and minerals, soybeans contain essential amino acids that can aid muscle repair and recovery. A study investigating the effects of soy supplementation on performance found that soy protein taken in combination with sago (a starchy source of carb) during moderate-intensity cycling delayed fatigue, resulting in an 84%

improvement in endurance (measured by time to exhaustion).

Citrus Fruits: It goes without saying that citrus fruits - orange, lemon, lime, and grapefruit- offer a potent dose of vitamin C. But did you know that these fruits also contain folate, which helps produce and maintain your body's cells, and fiber, which promotes GI health? Of course, vitamin C is the real star in this group, as it's critical for muscle and collagen repair –which can really come in handy if you're fighting off an injury or healing a wound.

Flaxseed: Flaxseed contains more inflammation-fighting Omega-3 than other readily available fat sources. Two components of flax, lignans and alpha-linolenic acid (ALA), have been found to assist immune health. Flaxseed is highly sensitive and easily oxidized, so for the most health benefit, purchase whole flaxseed and grind just before adding to your smoothie.

Noni Fruit: There are plenty of reasons that Noni fruit has gotten a lot of good press as of late. A host of research has found that Noni fruit (which is commonly sold in juice form) is a potent antioxidant that offers anti-inflammatory properties, cardiovascular boosters, and a host of other health benefits. A recent clinical trial found that the Noni supplementation resulted in a reduction in total cholesterol and triglycerides levels in subjects with both normal and elevated lipid levels (an indicator of heart disease) –and those benefits were even more significant for those subjects with elevated levels.

Oats: Not only are oats a tasty source of dietary fiber (1/4 cup of oat bran supplies nearly 4 grams), but beta-glucans, a component of the soluble fiber found in oats, has proven effective in lowering total blood cholesterol and low-density lipoprotein (LDL) levels –thus reducing your overall risk of heart disease. Added bonus? High fiber diets are more satiating, and have been linked to lower body weights. Try making a small batch of oatmeal and adding it to your next smoothie -you're likely to be pleasantly surprised by the thick shake that results. If you're not up for cooking, simply add oat bran instead.

Tomato: Tomatoes helps to prevent skin cancer due to its richness in lycopene. Lycopene also has been shown to promote prostate health. Add tomato to your next smoothie using either canned tomato that is whole or has been juiced – the nutrients in the tomato are concentrated and locked in during the canning process.

Coconut Water: The fat content in coconut water is extremely low, which means it can be consumed without the fear of immediately putting on the weight. It also helps to suppress appetite and make you feel less hungry because of coconut is very rich in nature. Coconut water aids in digestion as well. If you constantly encounter difficulty during digestion such as bloating or gastric pain, coconut water may provide an immediate source of relief. Coconut is high in fiber and this aids in preventing indigestion as well as reducing the occurrence of reflux.

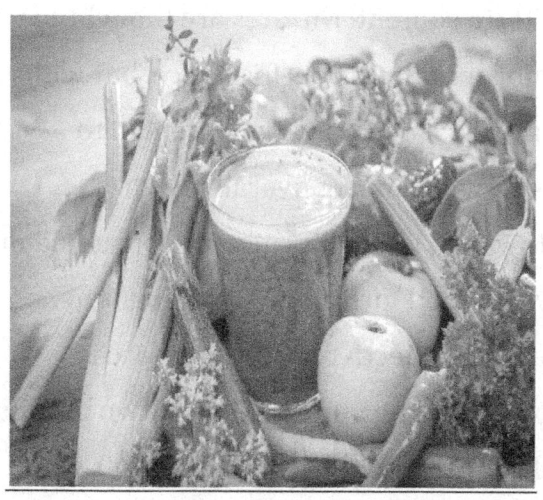

Vegetables:

Beets: Beets are getting a lot of press lately –mainly because of their high nitrate content. Nitrates are thought to improve athletic performance, but with a drawback of having the potential to negatively impact overall health. However, when nitrates are consumed in whole food form they are thought to be safe and effective. Recent research examined the performance of two groups of runners – one full of individuals who consumed baked beets before a 5K run, the second who took a placebo before running the same distance. The result? Individuals who consumed beets ran faster at the end of their runs, and also reported lower perceived exertion (meaning that even though they were running faster, it didn't feel harder).

Kale: Perhaps Popeye should've grabbed a can of kale instead of spinach. Kale is incredibly nutrient-dense, offering impressive amounts of potassium, as well as vitamins A, C, and K, in less than 35 calories. One cup of raw kale also packs potent amounts of antioxidants, notably lutein, which protects the eyes against oxidative damage and has been found to be effective in fighting macular degeneration.

Celery: Celery contains pthalides, which are organic chemical compounds that can lower the level of stress hormones in your blood. This allows your blood vessels to expand, giving your blood more room to move, and thereby reducing pressure.

Spinach: Exercise can increase your need for micronutrients like iron and zinc, and spinach is chock full of them. While low levels of iron and zinc can negatively impact athletic performance, cause fatigue, and even result in poor muscle growth, spinach delivers loads of these nutrients while also supplying folate, a B-vitamin responsible for producing and maintaining new cells. Folate is also essential for DNA and RNA production. Pregnant women and women seeking to become pregnant should be sure to take in adequate amounts of folate, as this micronutrient is essential for preventing neural tube defects.

Tea: Think outside the box and choose the most widely consumed beverage in the world (besides water) as a base for your next smoothie. Not only will you be adding flavor, you'll also get antioxidants, phytochemicals, and flavonoids –all of which fight oxidative damage and may reduce the risk of diseases like cancer and heart disease.

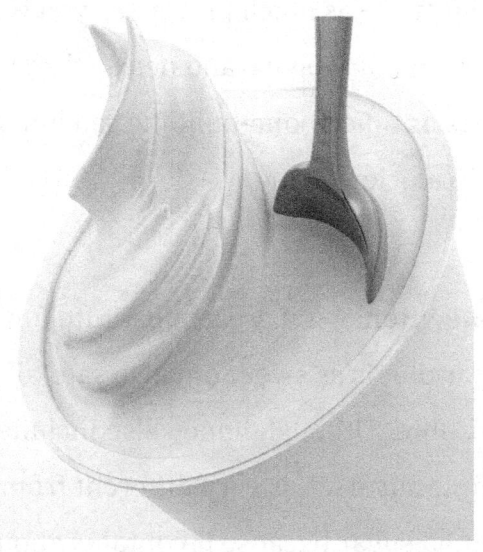

OTHERS

Greek Yogurt: Greek yogurt adds a calcium-packed protein boost to any smoothie. This popular snack item is thicker, creamier, and more nutrient-dense than traditional yogurts, and much like kefir, Greek yogurt contains probiotics that can boost GI and immune health. By going with Greek, you'll also get about twice as much protein as you would from regular yogurt, and nearly three times as much bone-building calcium per 150-calorie serving.

Honey: Honey is a great substitute for sugar that is as sweet but also safe to consume. Although honey also includes simple sugars, it is very different from refined sugar because it contains about

30% glucose and 40% fructose. Honey also helps reduce constipation, bloating and gas.

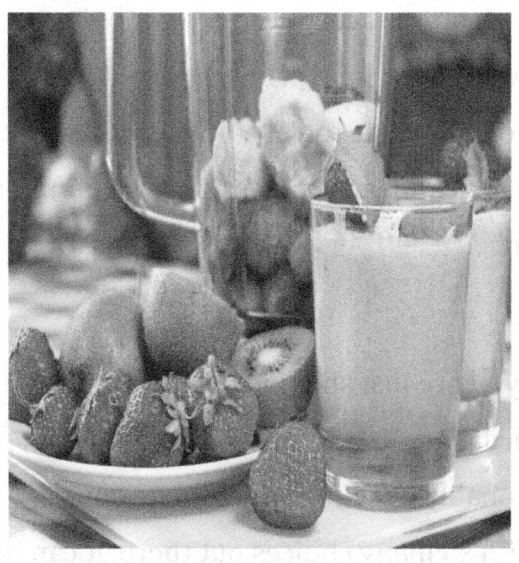

Equipment

Making smoothies should be easy and straightforward. There is no cooking involved, no long preparation – you should be able to get a nourishing snack or delicious meal in less than 10 minutes flat.

If you are just starting out, one of the hardest parts of making a smoothie is probably deciding which tools to use. With so many choices out there, it can be hard to navigate and decide on which tools you require.

In truth, there are only a few basic components that you will need in order to get your smoothie juice set up and running and let's go through them one by one!

1. Blender - This is the #1 tool that you need when attempting to make your own smoothies because the quality or type of blender will decide if your smoothie is a success. When choosing a blender, I always advocate going for the quality blender. They give the best consistency and best results. The reason is because you are probably going to use it very often if you have your mind set on the smoothie diet and a cheap blender is not going to cut it. The most important feature on any blender is a Pulse feature. Regardless of how many type of speeds you think you need, you will definitely be turning on the pulse feature more than anything else. Being able to pulse will give you greater control during blending to get your consistency just right.

2. Knives - The right knife for the job can make all the difference when you are trying to make your smoothies as efficiently as possible. We often use our knives to do necessary things like hull strawberries, quarter apples, chop chunky vegetables and split open plums and apricots to remove the pits. We also find ourselves reaching for our chef knives quite frequently; when we flash-freeze fruit in batches, a chef knife makes processing a big quantity of fruit a much simpler task, and you would be surprised at how many times we reach for our chef knife to chop a few nuts as a garnish for our smoothies! For choosing knives, I recommend having a paring knife and a chef's knife. Do look around your kitchen before you buy anything though – you might already have them lying around somewhere.

3. Measuring Cup and Spoon Set – This is a fairly straightforward decision. You just need a good set of measuring cup and spoon set to measure liquid and powdered ingredients. Something like this should be fairly inexpensive.

4. Silicone Spatulas – After you have blended your smoothie in the blender, you want to be able to get every single drop of it into your cup or bottle. Investing in a spatula is going to go a long way in achieving that purpose.

5. Beautiful Bottles or Glasses– This is where it matters more aesthetically than utility-wise. Once you have whipped up your mixture of goodness, you do not want to just drink it from the blender carriage (you can but where is the fun in that?). Prepare a beautiful glass and garnish the smoothie! Heck - show it to your family and friends and let them know that you are about to slurp up a glorious glass of goodness and lose a few pounds at the same time.

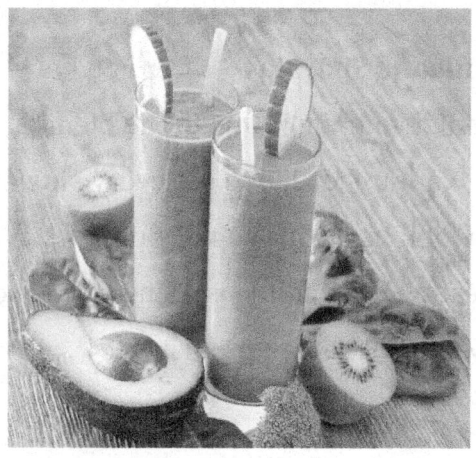

THINGS TO NOTE

Below is a list of things to note before you start the actual plan. It is important that you spend the time to go through this so that you properly understand how to process and prepare the smoothie.

- All ingredients should be raw. For the best results, I highly recommend using only leafy vegetables, fruits and water in the smoothies during the 10-day cleanse. You can, however, add in varying amounts of other ingredients as to your liking.

- Try to use dark leafy vegetables – they include beet greens, bokchoy, carrot top leaves, chard, arugula, dandelion greens, kale, mustard greens, parsley, radish tops, sorrel, spinach, watercress, spring greens, and turnip greens.

- Remove the stems of your greens for the best taste. Certain stems may give off a little bitter flavor which do not appeal to some people.

- Green smoothies can contain 40% greens are a source of protein. If you feel you need additional protein because of a heavy weights training or workout, you can add protein powder in your blender. Adding a scoop of protein powder to your smoothie everyday will also make you feel fuller for longer periods of time. It also helps keep your metabolism high and burn more calories. If you have to add protein powder, use a non-dairy, plant-based protein powder, such as rice, soy, or hemp protein, and not whey protein powder, which is made from cow's milk. I understand that this might be a little more difficult to purchase but the results should be well worth it.

- Use organic ingredients whenever possible. If you can't find organic fruits and vegetables, wash off the pesticides and waxes as best you can, using special cleansers from health food stores or vinegar, scrubbing and rinsing carefully.

- Use purified water in smoothies. Another option is to use alkaline water, which aids in detoxification and better hydration. You can add ice if you want. Tap water is not recommended for use.

- Add ample fruits. Fruits play an important role. For every smoothie meal, try to add in – banana, strawberries, blueberries, kiwi, pears are just a few examples of healthy fruits you can. Fruits also provide natural sweetening to your smoothie so that it tastes better. Always use ripe fruits to blend into your smoothies; if your fruits are unripe when you bought them, allow them to sit for a few days until they ripen. If you're diabetic or have candida, do not use high sugar level fruits (tropical fruits are usually high in sugar content). You definitely need to monitor your blood sugar, and get a doctor's permission before following the diet. Fruits that are low in sugar include lemons, limes, cherries, grapefruits, strawberries, cranberries, raspberries, goji berries, apples and blueberries. Fruits can be either used fresh or blended frozen. It is a common misconception that frozen fruits are not healthy; they are actually almost as nutritious as fresh ones.

- Ground flaxseeds are included in most recipes. Flaxseed contains Omega-3 essential fatty acids, lignans and excellent dietary fiber. Lignans have both plant estrogen and antioxidant qualities and Flaxseed contains up tp 75 to 800 times more lignans than other plant foods.

- Stevia is included in most recipes as a sweetener. Refined sugar is incredibly fattening, stevia is a 100% natural, zero calorie sweetener. On the contrary, Stevia lowers your blood sugar and help to fight diabetes.

Now that you have at least a fundamental knowledge of the things you need to prepare yourself with, it's time to head straight into the guide itself!

Chapter 3: Action Plan

This is where you will find the guide and instructions on the actual plan. Do read through this chapter carefully and understand what is required of the plan!

Many experts explain that the cleanse plan can to divided into two course of action.

1) Full Cleanse

2) Half Cleanse

Full cleanse involves only consuming smoothies, snacks, water and tea for the entire course of the smoothie plan. The full cleanse consists of three smoothies, snacks, and water/ tea for the entire ten days. This will provide the most health and weight-loss benefits, with an expected weight loss between ten to fifteen pounds.

The half cleanse is essentially the same as the full cleanse, however, for dinner, you consume actual solid food that is healthy. The key being that the dinner should not contain food that is counterproductive to yoursmoothie diet plan.

For the purposes of this book, we will only be going to the full cleanse plan, I'm a firm believer in staying committed to a goal and if this book go into too much detail on the half cleanse plan, it might just make you choose the easier way out. With that said, if at any point of time you are feeling unwell from only consuming smoothie, please feel free to switch to the half cleanse by eating solid food for dinner, or stop the smoothie diet completely.

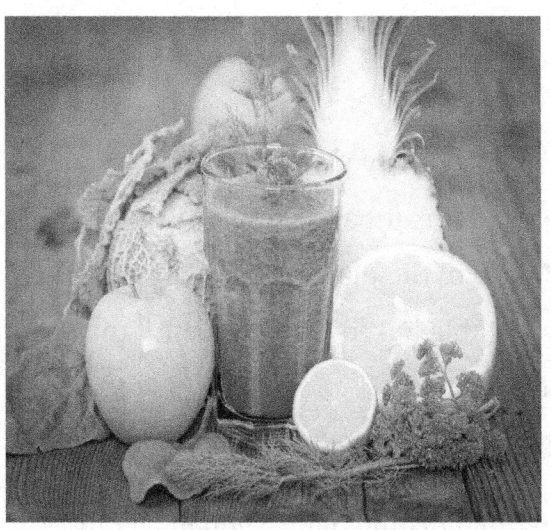

Instructions

Each day, you should drink up to 50 - 60 ounces of smoothies to ensure that you are properly nourished. The recipes in this book are designed for detoxification and weight loss. Each recipe for the cleanse plan is for 3 servings – they make about 33-48 ounces of smoothie, which you can divide into 3 servings of 11-16 ounces each.

For the 10 day plan, it is best for you to prepare fruit based smoothie for the first 2 days of the plan, followed by 8 days of vegetable based smoothie until the end of the cleanse.

In the morning before you head out, always remember to prepare your entire day worth of smoothies. Pack your smoothies and bring them with you.

Drink 1/3 of the smoothie every 4 hours throughout the day. If you are feeling hungry, sip on the smoothie until your hunger pang ceases.

Smoothie contains a lot of bubbles trapped in its thickened liquid, try to chew it as much as possible to avoid bloating.

Remember to use ONLY smoothies, not juices – smoothies contain whole foods with lots of fiber while juices don't. This has been discussed in the earlier chapters.

Some of you may not like the taste of your smoothie at first and not want to finish the entire day worth of smoothie. My advice to you is that you should at least finish 2/3 of the quantity to ensure that your body gets the minimum amount of nutrition. It is important to at least consume some smoothie or munch on a snack every 3-4 hours to keep the metabolism of your body amped up. Yes, you will desire to eat less food but you still need to feed your body with the fuel it needs every once in a while.

It is best to keep your smoothies as refrigerated as possible so that they do not oxidize too fast.

Blenders – Blenders have been discussed in the previous chapter. Overall, try to use a high-speed blender, around 1000 watts. A few of the more well-known brands are: Vitamix, Blendtec, andNutribullet.

Fat blasting smoothies

Snacking on apples (not too many though), celery, carrots, cucumbers, and other crunchy veggies throughout the day is acceptable. You may also snack on other high protein snacks in moderation and they include unsweetened peanut butter, hard-boiled eggs, raw nuts and seeds (only a handful).

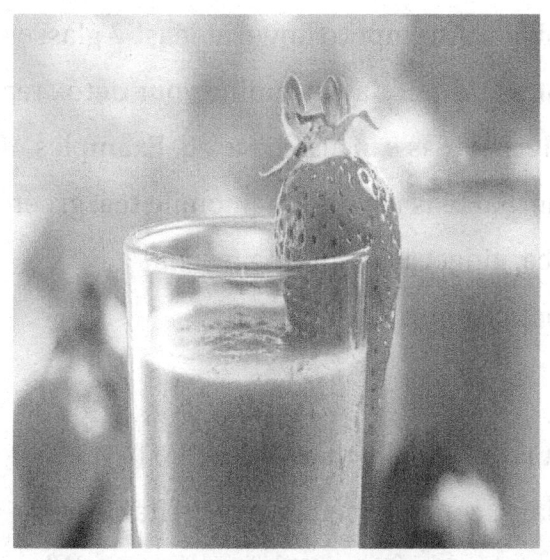

Daily routine

Every morning, you should start by drinking a few glasses of water to replenish your body fluid. About 15 minutes after, drink some detox tea that will provide cleansing support for your kidneys and livers. Consistent hydration is very important during the cleansing phase. Attempt to down at least 7 glasses of water per day including your detox tea. Herbal teas can also be used. Examples of herbal teas include chamomile tea, green tea, ginger tea, Ginseng tea and peppermint tea.

It is very likely that within the first few days, you will feel hungry, irritable and experience frequent hunger pangs. When you are undergoing these phases, you may snack gently.

To ensure that the side effects of smoothie cleanse do not affect your day-to-day activities, it is recommended that you start it on a weekend rather than on a Monday. This will at least give you 2 days to get used to it before heading out for work the following week.

Typical detoxification symptoms include pains, nausea, cravings, headaches,lethargy, muscle aches, skin rashes, and irritability. If the detox symptoms prolong and do not go away after 1-2 days, try to do the following:

1) Use higher proportion of fruits in your smoothie ingredients for the first few days and gradually switch up the ratio of vegetable accordingly over the next few

days. Fruits are generally more acceptable by our body than raw vegetable.

2) Drink lots of water to keep your body hydrated.

3) Start the cleanse gradually – on your first day, have a smoothie for breakfast and eat light, healthy meals for lunch and dinner (big salads). Remember to still avoid sugar, meats, dairy, etc. On your second day, have green smoothies for breakfast and lunch but a light healthy meal, such as a salad, for dinner. By the third day, you should be ready to resume with green smoothies all day. If not, just switch to the modified cleanse for the remainder of the cleanse period.

Chapter 4: Fruit-based Smoothies

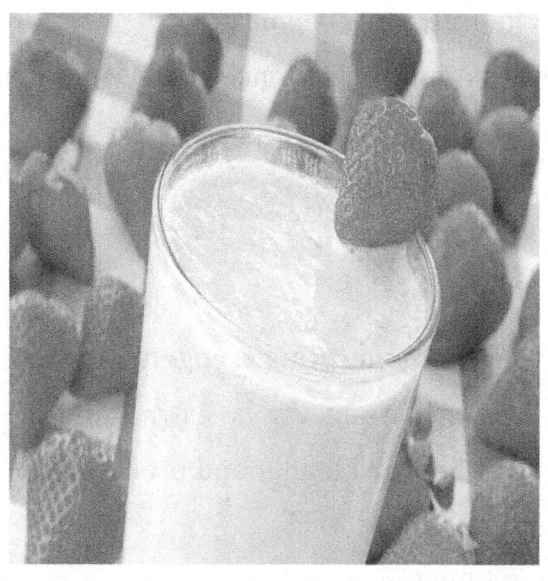

Fruit based smoothies are a great way to start the cleansing because your body is more adapted to absorbing fruits than raw greens. Here, you will find some great fruit based recipes that are both delicious and nourishing!

1. Orange Wonderland
Servings: 3
3 navel orange, peeled
¾ fat free greek yoghurt
6tbsp orange juice concentrate (omit if do not wish to consume sugar)
3/4 tsp vanilla extract
12 ice cubes

Steps: Combine orange, yoghurt, orange juice concentrate, vanilla extract and ice cubes. Pour in blender and process until smooth.
Nutrition (per serving): 160 cal
Best for: Cooling down on a hot workout day. Low calories and packed with vitamin C.

2. Blueberry Banana Tea

Servings: 3

9 tbsp water

2 green tea bag

6 tbsp honey

4 ½ cup frozen blueberries

1 ½ medium banana

2 cup soy milk

Steps: Microwave water on high until steaming hot in a cup or bowl. Place tea bags in water and let tea brew for 3-5 minutes. Remove tea bags and add honey into tea until completely dissolved. Combine milk, banana and berries in a blender. Add tea to blender. Process the mixture on high setting until it is smooth. If smoothie becomes dry, add ¼ cup of water. Pour and serve.

Nutrition: 269 cal

Best for: Antioxidant and extremely nutritious. Makes for a good meal.

3. Berry Berry Smoothie
Servings: 3
2 cup frozen strawberries
2 cup frozen blueberries
2 ½ almond milk
½ cup frozen raspberries
3 tbsp honey
2 tbsp grated ginger
3 tbsp flaxseed
6 tbsp lemon juice

Steps: Combine all ingredients in blender, add lemon juice according to taste. Process until smooth and pour into chilled glass or bottle
Nutrition: 112 cal

Best for: Packed with vitamin c and start the day with a bang.

4. Tomato Yoghurt Smoothie

Servings: 3

3 cups low-fat plain yoghurt
2 large ripe plum or round tomatoes, peeled, seeded and chopped
1 ½ tsp dried basil
1 ½ tsp salt cherry tomatoes and ice, to serve (optional)

Steps: In a blender, combine yoghurt, tomatoes, basil and salt until very smooth Serve over ice and garnish with cherry tomatoes.

Nutrition: 88 cal

Best for: Hearty filling tomato based smoothie. Super low in calories.

5. Mango Delight

Servings: 3

3 ripe mangoes

1 cup greek yoghurt

600ml skim milk, chilled

1 tsp honey

2 tbsp chia seed

Steps: Peel the mango and remove flesh away from the core. Place flesh in a blender and pulse. Pour in yoghurt and milk. Process mixture until smooth. Add honey to taste. Pour in to glasses and serve.

Nutrition: 158 cal

Best for: Sweet and low calorie meal, satisfies your craving for sugar if you are on the verge of giving up!

5. Chocolate Blueberry Smoothie

Servings: 3

6 cups spinach

3 cup blueberries, frozen

3 scoop chocolate protein powder

6tbsp dark cocoa powder

1 ½ cup unsweetened almond milk

Steps: Roughly chop spinach, combine all into blender and blitz until smooth texture. Pour and serve.

Nutrition: 124 cal

Best for: Spinach provides a healthy amount of iron and fiber, the chocolate and blueberries pumps your body up with antioxidants.

6. Pomegranate Berry Goodness

Servings: 3

3 cup pomegranate juice (fresh or juiced)

3 cup silken tofu

6 cups assorted berries, frozen

4tbsp honey

Steps: Peel pomegranate and remove seed. Press seed to extract juices until cup is filled. Pour juice, tofu and berries into blender and process until smooth. Add honey to taste.

Nutrition: 109 cal

Best for: Pomegranate contains high levels of antioxidant and tofu gives you the necessary protein and calcium.

7. Berry Lemonade

Servings: 3

1 ½ cup fresh strawberries

3 large date, pitted

1 ½ cup unsweetened almond milk

3 tbsp raw cashews

5 tbsp fresh lemon juice

1 ½ teaspoon finely grated lemon zest

6 ice cubes (Optional, can be replaced with half cup water)

Steps: Combine ingredientsinto blender and pulse. Blitz until smooth texture.

Nutrition: 178 cal

Best for: Refreshing drink that is also an ultimate thirst quencher. Packed with vitamin C, provides a sweet getaway without the actual sugary guilt.

8. The Safe Mojito

Servings: 3

1 cup coconut water

2 tbsp hemp seeds

½-1 tsp spirulina (optional)

2 tbsp freshly squeezed limejuice

½ avocado

1 frozen banana

2 dates, pitted

1 handful fresh mint leaves

Steps: There is no alcohol here. Slice lime and squeeze out juice. Add all ingredients into blender and blitz. Pour out mixture and add additional mint leaves for garnish

Nutrition: 172 cal

Best for: Good source of protein as well as nutrients like B complex vitamins, that help turn out food into energy.

CHAPTER 5: VEGETABLE BASED SMOOTHIES

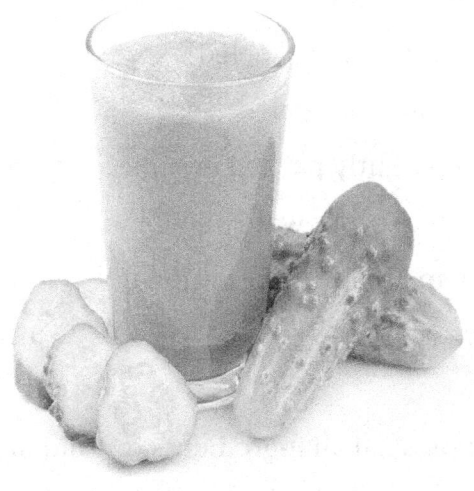

This is the real deal of green smoothies. Vegetable based smoothie helps to cleanse your palate and makes the most fiber and minerals you need to detoxify your body.

1. Spinach orange smoothie

Servings: 3

Ingredients:
3 navel orange, peeled
1 ½ banana, peeled
6 cup tightly packed organic spinach
1 cup coconut water, adjusted as desired
1 tbsp hemp seeds, optional
Ice

Steps: Add all ingredients to a blender with a few ice cubes and blend on high to combine. Add more coconut water as desired to reach desired consistency for smoothie. Pour into a glass and enjoy!

Nutrition: 120 cal

2. Blueberry Mint Green Smoothie

Servings: 3

6 cups spinach

6 cups blueberry (I used 1 c. fresh and 1 c. frozen)

3 kiwi

Handful large mint leaves

3 cup coconut water

2 cup ice

Steps: Put all ingredients in a blender and mix it up!

Nutrition: 144 cal

3. Spring Detox Smoothie

Servings: 3

3 cup green tea, chilled

3 tablespoon fresh ginger, grated

3 cup loosely packed cilantro

2 avocado

4 cup loosely packed organic baby kale (or another baby green)

3 cup cucumber

3 cup pineapple

2 lemon

Steps:Squeeze juice of 1 lemon. Place lemon and rest of ingredients into a blender and puree until smooth. Nutrition: 171 cal

4. Popeye Shake

Servings: 3

1/2 banana

3/4 cup milk

2 big handfuls spinach

1/4 cup raw rolled oats

1/2 scoop protein powder

Fat blasting smoothies

1 tbsp flax
Granola topping

Steps: Roughly chop spinach leaves, add all ingredients into blender and blitz until smooth.

Nutrition: 120 cal

5. Coconut Honeydew Mint Smoothie
Servings: 3

1/2 honeydew melon, cut into chunks (about 4 cups, or 1 1/2 lbs)
1/2 cup light coconut milk
1-2 leaves fresh mint (plus more for garnish)
1/2-1 tsp fresh lime juice (or to taste)
1 cup ice

Drizzle of honey or coconut nectar, to taste (optional, depending on how sweet your melon is)

Steps:Cut your melon in half, remove the seeds, and slice away the outer rind. Cut the melon into chunks, and add to your blender along with the coconut milk, mint, lime, and ice. Blend until smooth. Taste, and adjust sweetness with honey or coconut nectar. Serve with a garnish of mint, or fresh melon slices.

Nutrition: 143 cal

6. Peachy Green Protein
Servings: 3
2 scoops protein powder
1 cup unsweetened almond milk

1 cup frozen peaches

1/2 cup frozen pineapple

1/2 banana

2 cups kale

1 tbsp ground flaxseed

Steps: Add all ingredients to blender. Mix until smooth.

Nutrition: 120 cal

7. Coffee Peanut Drink

Servings: 3

3/4 cup whole milk

1/4 cup strong espresso, slightly cooled

1/2 cup frozen banana

1/4 cup smooth peanut butter

1/4 cup dark chocolate, roughly chopped

Ice, as needed

agave syrup, optional to sweeten

Steps:

Pour milk and espresso into blender jar. Add frozen banana, peanut butter and half cup of ice. Cover with lid and process until smooth.

Taste smoothie and add agave syrup as needed to sweeten. Add additional ice if thicker consistency is desired. Add chopped dark chocolate and pulse for a couple seconds until chocolate bits are distributed (and added ice is blended). Serve immediately.

Nutrition: 180 cal

8. Tropical Protein Smoothie
Servings: 3

1 cup unsweetened vanilla almond milk

3 large handful kale (the leaves of about 8 stalks)
2/3 cup pineapple chunks
1 ripe avocado
2 scoop protein powder (i used vanilla)
1 c ice cubes

Steps: Combine all ingredients into a blender and puree until smooth!
Nutrition: 135 cal

9. Coconut Green Smoothie
Servings: 3

5 cups fresh spinach
5 cups almond milk, unsweetened
3 large apple, cored, any variety
2 banana

1 cup rolled oats

2 tbsp coconut oil

1 ½ tsp ground cinnamon

Steps: Blend spinach and almond milk until smooth. Add remaining ingredients, and blend until smooth.

Nutrition: 137 cal

Chapter 6: Energizing Smoothies

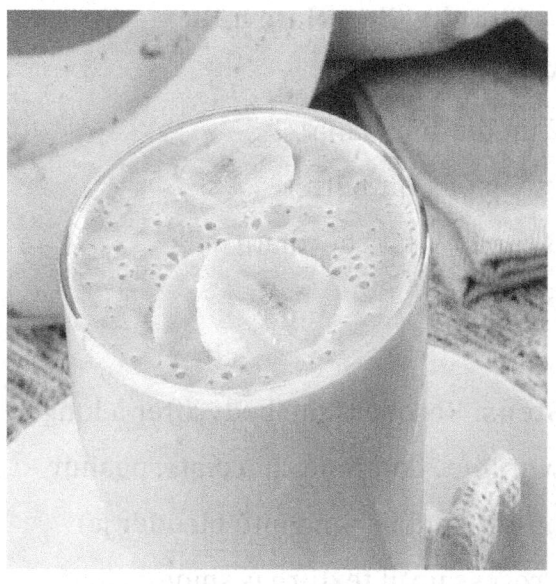

Over here, you will find an extensive list of smoothies that will provide you with good amounts of energy replenishment that keeps you active throughout the day! The best time to drink energizing smoothies is after a long work out or in the evening after work.

1. Chunky Chocolate milk
Servings: 3

2 medium banana

3tbsp peanut butter

3 cup low-fat chocolate milk

6 ice cubes

Steps: Recovers the body after a long workout. Combine chocolate, peanut butter, and banana into blender jar. Process until texture is smooth. Serve immediately.

Nutrition: 160 cal

2. Cantaloupe Yoghurt

Servings: 3

½ cantaloupe, seeded and roughly chopped

½ cup plain Greek yogurt

1 tbsp honey

3 ice cubes

Steps:

This smoothie has a whole half of a cantaloupe (superfood alert!), which helps hydrate after a sweaty workout (since it's 89 percent water). Plus, one cup of the fruit has as much potassium as a medium banana!

Nutrition: 148 cal

3. Cinnamon Sweet Potato

Servings: 3

3tsp cinnamon powder

2 scoop whey protein

¾ cup sweet potato

3 cup vanilla almond milk

6 ice cubes

Steps: Boil sweet potato until cooked and dice in cubes. Place all ingredients into blender and process until smooth. Pour into glass and serve. This recipe is packed with protein and can replenish glycogen stores after an intense workout session.

Nutrition: 171 cal

4. Tofu Cherry Energizer

Servings: 3

2 cup water

4 bags rooibos tea

15 ounces silken tofu

6 cups sweet cherries, frozen

3 cup grapes, frozen

1 ½ cup blueberries, frozen

Steps: Microwave water in bowl until steaming hot. Place tea bags in hot water and let brew for 5 minutes. Remove tea bags. Place all ingredients into blender and add in the hot tea last. Process until mixture becomes smooth. Pour and serve. Tofu thickens the smoothie as well as adding protein. Red tea adds antioxidants and cherries help with muscle recovery. Overall, this is a great energy boosting drink!

Nutrition: 164 cal

5. Twist of Taste
Servings: 3

15 ounces carrot juice
1 ½ cup avocado
3tbsp fresh lemon juice
1/2 cup water
3tbsp freshly grated ginger
2 inch of cayenne pepper (or 3 scoops of powder)

Steps: Grate ginger finely and add all ingredients into blender. Process until smooth and serve. This drink tastes zingy and savory. It contains cayenne pepper which is known to curb appetite and boost metabolism.

Nutrition: 109 cal

6. Fruity Oatmeal

Servings: 3

1 ¼ cup orange juice

6 peach slices, frozen (or about half a peach)

12 strawberries, frozen

¾ cup rolled oats

1 cup plain, fat-free Greek yogurt

2tbsp chia seeds

5 ice cubes

Steps: De-core and slice peach. Microwave 1 bowl water and cook oats in hot water for 3 minutes until mixture becomes thick and paste–like. Combine all ingredient into blender and pulse. This mix is thick due to the oats and yoghurt. Process until chunks are broken down and serve. Add water if mixture becomes too thick.

Nutrition: 168 cal

7. Pina Colada

Servings: 3

½ cup unsweetened almond milk

½ cup coconut water

1 tbsp shredded coconut flesh

¼ tsp vanilla extract

½ cup pineapple, frozen

1 tsp honey

Steps: Open coconut and remove flesh with spoon (or buy ready-made coconut flesh). Combine ingredients in blender and process until smooth. This smoothie includes pineapple, which boosts the immune system and has a ton of vitamin C.

Nutrition: 158 cal

8. Spices Raspberry

Servings: 3

2 cup water

3 banana

1 tsp turmeric

1 tsp cinnamon

5 stalks collard greens

1 cup raspberries, frozen

4 tbsp hemp seeds

Steps: Slice banana into chunk. Roughly chop collard greens. Combine ingredients into blender and process until smooth. Curcumin is the main active ingredient in turmeric. It has powerful anti-inflammatory effects and is a very strong antioxidant.

Nutrition: 112 cal

9. Almond Creamy Shake

Servings: 3

2 cup almond milk

5 tbsp Greek yogurt

1 scoop vanilla protein powder

1 ½ tsp vanilla extract

3 ice cubes

3 tbsp almond butter

1 ½ banana, frozen

3 tbsp jam

Steps: Break banana into blender and add in rest of ingredients. Process until smooth and serve.

Nutrition: 179 cal

Chapter 7: Breakfast Smoothies

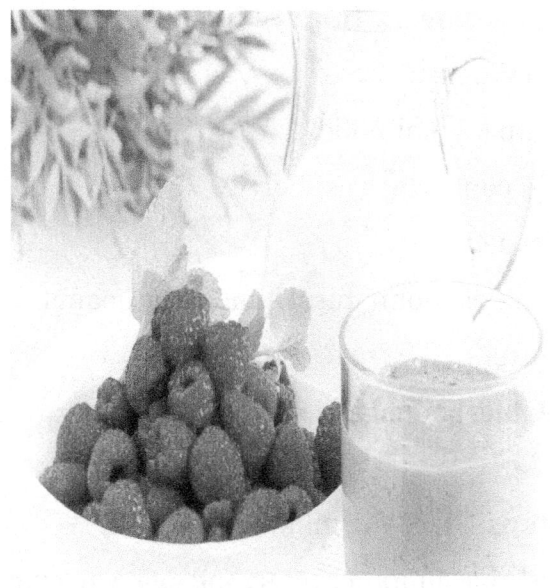

Breakfast provides the body and brain with supplements and fuel that is required after an overnight fast. Without breakfast, you are effectively running on an empty tank and it's going to make you feel lethargic throughout the day. Here are some yummy, hearty recipes that will help to kick start your day nicely!

1) Raspberry Honey Milk
Servings: 3
2cup low-fat milk
2½ cupfrozen raspberries
2banana
3 tablespoonnatural almond or peanut butter
3tablespoonagave nectar or honey

Steps: Place the milk, raspberries, banana, almond butter, and agave nectar in a blender.Blend until smooth and frothy.

Nutrition: 181 cal

2) Ginger Berry Oatmeal

Servings: 3

¾ cup old-fashioned rolled oats

2 cup frozen blueberries

1½ cup plain low-fat yogurt

1½ cup ice

4 tbsp brown sugar

¾ tsp grated fresh ginger

Steps:Place the oats and ½ cup of water in a blender.Let oat soak until the oats have softened. This should take about 15 minutes.Add the blueberries, yogurt, ice, sugar and ginger.Process until smooth.

Nutrition: 145 cal

3) Tropical Green Detox

Servings: 3

1 ½ cup coconut milk

5 cups stemmed and chopped kale or spinach

3 cups chopped pineapple (about 1/4 medium pineapple)

3 ripe banana, chopped

Steps: Combine the coconut milk, ½ cup water, the kale, pineapple, and banana in a blender and puree until smooth. This will take about 1 minute, adding more water to reach the desired consistency.

Nutrition: 101 cal

4) Mango Milkshake

Servings: 3

3cup chopped ripe mango

2cup low-fat milk

1 ½ cup ice

¾cup plain low-fat yogurt

3tbsp honey

Steps: Skin mango and remove flesh from core. Place the mango, milk, ice, yogurt, and honey in a blender. Blend until smooth and frothy.

5) Pomegranate Booster

Servings: 3

1 cup pomegranate Juice

3/4 cup soy or low-fat milk

2 ice cubes

1 large banana

2 tbsp almonds

3 tbsp protein powder (optional)

1 tsp honey or stevia sweetener

Steps: In a blender combine all ingredients. Cover and blend on high for at least 30 seconds (make sure the almonds aren't visible) then pour into two glasses.

Nutrition: 183 cal

6) Coffee Banana Smoothie

Servings: 3

3 sliced peeled banana

1 cup low-fat milk

1/2 cupcold black coffee,

2 tsp sugar

1/2 cup ice in a blender.

Steps: Brew coffee and place in fridge to chill. Combine cold coffee, banana, milk and sugar in blender and process until smooth.

Nutrition: 170 cal

7) Raspberry Date Shake
Servings: 3
2 cups water
3tbsp flax seeds
5 bananas
4 cups frozen raspberries (260 grams)
10 dates (de-seeded)

Steps: Peel dates and ensure that seeds are removed. Combine all the ingredients in a blender and process until smooth.

Nutrition: 136 cal

8) Strawberry Orange Blend

Servings: 3

8 cups ripe strawberries

3 cup plain yogurt

1 ½ cup fresh orange juice

2tbsp sugar

8 thin orange slices (optional)

Steps: Hull the strawberries and add the hulled strawberries to a food processor or blender. Add the yogurt, orange juice, and sugar. Process the mixture on the highest speed until a well-blended puree forms. This should last about 15 seconds. Stop to scrape down the sides of the container once or twice. Pour into glass and serve.

Nutrition: 146 cal

9) Apple Oat Smoothie

Servings: 3

3 apples, peeled, cored, cubed

1 cup rolled oats

1 1/2 cup rice milk

2tsp honey or agave

1/2tsp cinnamon

Steps: Soak oats in rice milk for 5 minutes. (Or add oat to hot water for a thicker mixture) Combine all ingredients in blender. Process until well blended.

Nutrition: 139 cal

CHAPTER 8: QUICK SMOOTHIES

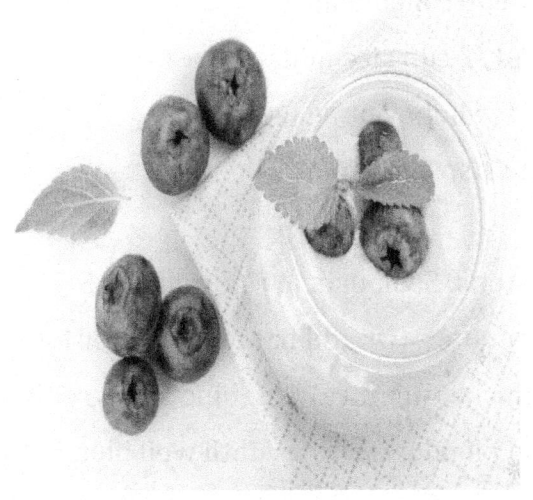

Here are a bunch of recipes are that are blazing fast to make. No slicing, no cutting – simply chuck them down the blender, process and you are good to go! This is great for the "busy bees" who are running tight on time. Most of the recipes you see here will have no more than 5 ingredients and yet, taste delicious and nutritious!

1) Raspberry Coconut Cocoa

Servings: 3

3 cup unsweetened coconut milk (from a carton)
2 cup frozen raspberries
4 scoops protein shake
3tbsp chia seeds
3tbsp white chocolate chips
4tbsp water

Steps: In a blender, mix all ingredients until smooth.

Nutrition: 120 cal

2) Berry Honey Tea

Servings: 3

1 ½ cup frozen blueberries

5 cups green tea, room temperature

3tbsp agave nectar

Steps: Divide blueberries between compartments of an ice cube tray. Fill with green tea and freeze. Puree in blender with remaining green tea and agave.

Nutrition: 126 cal

3) Berry Pomegranate Mix

Servings: 3

6 cups mixed frozen berries

3 cup unsweetened pomegranate juice

2 cup water

Steps: Combine all ingredients in a blender, and blend until smooth.

Nutrition: 87 cal

4) Simple Berries Delight

Servings: 3

6 navel oranges, peel and pith removed, cut into chunks
2 cup frozen blueberries
2 cup frozen raspberries

Steps: Combine all ingredients in a blender, and blend until smooth.

Nutrition: 101 cal

5) Summer Tofu Smoothie

Servings: 3

1 ½ cup silken tofu

3 ripe banana

5 cup frozen mixed berries

1 ½ cup fresh orange juice

Steps: Combine all ingredients in a blender, and blend until smooth.

Nutrition: 117 cal

6) Strawberry Banana Milkshake

Servings: 3

3 ripe banana

6 cups frozen strawberries (8 ounces)

3 cup soy milk

4tbsp honey

Steps: Combine all ingredients in a blender, and blend until smooth.

Nutrition: 106 cal

7) Blueberry Banana Yoghurt
Servings: 3

3 ripe banana

3 cups frozen blueberries

2 cup plain low-fat yogurt

4tbsp honey

Steps: Combine all ingredients in a blender, and blend until smooth.

Nutrition: 123 cal

8) Blackberry Wheat Smoothie

Servings: 3

3 ripe banana

3 cups frozen blackberries (8 oz.)

2 cup fresh orange juice

4tbsp toasted wheat germ

Steps: Combine all ingredients in a blender, and blend until smooth.

Nutrition: 135 cal

9) Green Tart Smoothie

Servings: 3

5 cups fresh kale

3 cup water

5 large stalks of celery, chopped

1 ½ cucumber, chopped

Fat blasting smoothies

1 ⅓ grapefruit
3 cup frozen pineapple

Steps: Blend kale and water until smooth. Add remaining ingredients, and blend until smooth.

Nutrition: 90 cal

Conclusion

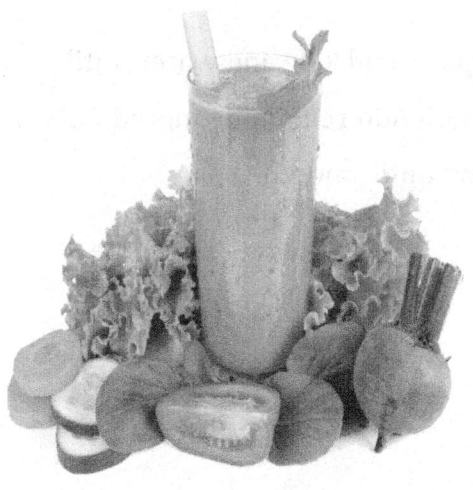

I hope you have gained a much better understanding on the 10 day cleanse plan! Smoothie cleanse have picked up popularity of late. It is well-known for being one of the easier and healthier way of losing weight in a short period of time. No more chasing the next magic pill and weight loss drug. I'm a living product of the 10-daycleanse and I've since led a much healthier lifestyle than before. I consistently feel great and look forward to my daily workouts.

To maximize the potential of this cleansing plan, throw in some cardio exercise! Try to run 15-30minutes a day and you will see the results almost improve drastically.The plan has worked very well for me and I firmly believe that it can do wonders for you as well!

If you have noticed, the smoothies are actually not difficult to make at all. Most of them involve simply chugging the ingredients into a blender and processing the mixture. The difficult thing to do is to really stay committed to the plan and seeing out the entire full cleanse. Raw vegetable smoothies do not go down easy for everybody and it is rather disheartening to see a lot people give up before seeing any results. Weight loss results may vary slightly for different people, but one should not judge the success of this plan based solely on the numerical figure of the amount of weight loss. I lost more than 15 pounds, but this is because I quite overweight at the point of time. If you are underweight, know that there is simply no way you can lose 15 pounds!

Besides weight loss, you are also undergoing a complete detoxification of your body, as well as switching your lifestyle for the better. Achieving these two targets is already a pretty decent result; so do not be discouraged by the fact that you have not lost enough weight.

Finally, smoothie diet should be fun! Many people including myself find the process of creating smoothies to be rather enjoyable. You can think of yourself as a modern day chemist, mixing and matching different ingredients to concoct your very own potion. If you have kids or significant other, this is also a great way to share the fun with them. Make easy-to-prepare smoothies with them and let them choose the ingredients! You might not be able to get your kids to eat a big bowl of kale, but when they are not looking, quietly chug a bunch into a berry smoothie, and they probably won't even notice!

Enjoy this entire process and I sincerely hope that you will join me on the other side of the cleanse plan! Stay happy, stay blissful.

Made in the USA
Monee, IL
04 May 2025